The COLLAGEN Diet Cookbook

A Planned Program to Help You Lose Weight, Prevent Disease, Improve Digestion and Renew your Youth in 28-Day.

By

Kim Cox

The Collagen Diet Cookbook

Copyright © 2019, By: *Kim Cox*

ISBN: 978-1-950772-20-9

All Rights Reserved. No part of this publication may be reproduced in any form or by any means, including scanning, photocopying, or otherwise without prior written permission of the copyright holder.

Disclaimer:

The information provided in this book is designed to provide helpful information on the subjects discussed. The publisher and author are not responsible for any specific health or allergy needs that may require medical supervision and are not liable for any damages or negative consequences from any treatment, action, application or preparation, to any person reading or following the information in this book.

The Collagen Diet Cookbook

Table of Contents

- INTRODUCTION: 6
  - The Collagen Diet 6
- **COLLAGEN BONE BROTH RECIPES** 7
  - Slow Cooker Beef Barbacoa 7
  - Slow Cooked Beef Bourguignon 9
  - Salsa de Guajillo 12
  - Chicken Mushroom Risotto 13
  - Easy New Orleans Slow Cooker Shrimp Jambalaya 15
  - Healthy Greek Quinoa Salad with Simple Lemon Dressing 17
  - Slow Cooker Curry Chicken 19
  - Creamy Mushroom Pasta 22
  - Southern Collard Greens with Bone Broth 24
  - Turkey Pot Pie 26
  - Slow Cooker Split Pea Soup 28
  - French Onion Soup 30
  - Cream of Chicken Soup Recipe 32
  - White Bean Chili 34
  - Chicken Tortilla Soup 36
  - Salsa Verde Recipe 39
  - Red White and Blue Kansas-City Style BBQ Bone Broth 40
  - Veggie-Packed Dairy-Free Creamy Broccoli Soup 41
  - Slow Cooker Chicken Bone Broth Recipe 43
  - Bone Broth Gazpacho Recipe with Cilantro Chimichurri 45
- **COLLAGEN GLUTEN FREE RECIPES** 48
  - Creamy Tomato Soup with Coconut and Curry 48
  - Creamy Potato Leek Soup 50

Creamy Asparagus Soup with Avocado and Fennel 52

Black Bean Soup with Smoked Paprika and Chipotle 54

Paleo Butternut Squash Soup 56

Slow Cooker Creamy Sweet Potato Soup with Coconut and Pistachios 59

Lentil Soup with Mushroom Chicken Bone Broth 61

COLLAGEN GUT-FRIENDLY RECIPES 63

Pesto Zucchini Pasta (Whole 30 Approved) 63

Quinoa Buddha Breakfast Bowl 65

Baked Almond-Crusted Cod with Sautéed Bok Choy and Bell Peppers 67

Bone Broth Ice Cubes 69

Coconut Vegetable Curry Over Quinoa 71

Sweet Potato Toast (Whole30 Approved) 73

Wholesome Cabbage Soup with Spicy Kimchi 75

COLLAGEN KETO RECIPES 77

Korean Keto Meatballs 77

Loaded Cauliflower Keto Soup 79

Creamy Keto Mushroom Soup 81

Instant Pot Spicy Creamy Keto Chicken Soup 83

Homemade Keto Eggnog 85

Keto Fat Bombs with Cacao and Cashew 87

Keto Broccoli Cheese Soup 89

Keto Brussels Sprouts Gratin 91

Keto Pizza with Pepperoni 93

Baked Almond-Crusted Cod with Sautéed Bok Choy and Bell Peppers 95

Keto Overnight Oats with Coconut and Blueberries 98

The Best Keto Meatloaf 99

Keto Fried Chicken 101

COLLAGEN SMOOTHIE AND SHAKES 103

Creamy Chocolate Collagen Smoothie 103

The Collagen Diet Cookbook

Blueberry Explosion Collagen Smoothie 104

Chocolate Almond Butter Collagen Shake 105

Chocolate Peppermint Collagen Smoothie 106

Chocolate Peppermint Collagen Smoothie 107

Acai Superfood Collagen Smoothie 108

German Chocolate Cake Collagen Smoothie 109

Chocolate Mint Shake 110

Best Keto Collagen Peptide Smoothie Ever (Easy Recipe) 111

Strawberry Moringa Mint Smoothie 112

Blueberry Muffin Smoothie Bowl Healthy Recipe 113

Blueberry Muffin Smoothie Bowl 114

Apple Banana Smoothie 115

Raw Superfood Smoothie 117

Steamed Spinach Smoothie "Pucks" 118

Roasted Strawberry Protein Smoothie 119

Keto Smoothie - Blueberry 121

Happy Digestion Smoothie 122

Kale Blueberry Smoothie 124

Better Than Botox Green Smoothie 125

Blueberry Granola Power Smoothie 126

Keto Chocolate Smoothie 127

Banana Chocolate Collagen Shake 128

Blueberry Collagen Smoothie 129

Blueberry Collagen Smoothie (Glowing Skin!) 130

COOL AS A CUCUMBER SMOOTHIE 131

THE BRAZILIAN FACE-LIFT 132

ISLAND TIME SHIFTER 133

INTRODUCTION:

The Collagen Diet

Collagen is a special type of protein found in the connective tissue and bones of humans and animals. It provides support and structure to the body, particularly the skin, ligaments, tendons, muscles, and skeletal system. Primarily collagen is made from the amino acids Glycine, Proline, and Hydroxyproline. The body produces its own collagen from free amino acids, but this process slows down as one age. This natural decrease in collagen production plays a role in the development of many common age-related concerns, like wrinkling of the skin, and joint pain and bone loss associated with osteoarthritis and osteoporosis, respectively.

However, collagen is one of the latest buzzwords in health. It's difficult to escape a grocery store without seeing tubs of powdered collagen or browse in a drugstore without noticing creams that claim they'll boost collagen to keep you looking young and youthful for decades to come. It's true that this protein plays an essential role in the perceived youthfulness of your skin, but there's more to it. "Collagen is a protein and is one of the major building blocks of our skin.

Nutrition plays a major role! By consuming a healthy balanced diet, you can get an adequate supply of amino acids to improve the natural production of collagen in your body. The protein can be derived from a variety of sources and the best way is to eat products loaded with minerals, vitamins, and antioxidants like bone broth, egg whites, nuts, grains, chicken, oily fish, cheese, beans, chia seeds, and leafy, green vegetables etc.

Nevertheless, as we grow older, we'll start to notice that our skin isn't as supple as before and is more prone to sagging. That's because the production of collagen in the body, the foundation of connective tissue that supports the skin structure, slows down gradually when we turn 35. Free radicals, exposure to the sun, and pollution also disintegrates collagen, which is why our skin starts forming wrinkles and thin with age.

Choosing to eat collagen-rich food can help to reverse the effects of aging skin. Make sure you include these foods into your daily diet to achieve younger-looking skin you'll love waking up to!

COLLAGEN BONE BROTH RECIPES

Slow Cooker Beef Barbacoa

Course Main Course

Prep Time 5 minutes

Cook Time 8 hours

Servings 8

Ingredients

- 1 medium onion (sliced)
- 1 cup of Kettle and Fire Beef Bone Broth
- 1 ½ tablespoons of ground cumin
- 2 teaspoons of salt
- ¼ teaspoon of ground cloves
- 3 bay leaves
- 3-4 pounds of beef chuck roast
- 3-4 chipotle peppers in adobo sauce
- 4 cloves garlic
- 1 tablespoon of dried oregano
- ½ teaspoon of ground black pepper
- ¼ cup of fresh lime juice

Ingredients for Serving:

Chopped white onion

Chopped avocado

Tortillas

Chopped tomatoes

Chopped fresh cilantro

Directions:

1. First, you cut beef into large cubes and place them in a slow cooker, then add onions.
2. After which you place chipotle peppers, garlic, oregano, pepper, bone broth, cumin, salt, ground cloves, and lime juice in a food processor.
3. After that, pulse until blended.
4. Then you pour the mixture over the beef (make sure you add bay leaves).
5. At this point, cover and cook on low for about 8-9 hours or on high for 6 hours.
6. This is when you shred the beef with two forks.
7. Finally, use tongs to serve the barbacoa in tortillas with your desired toppings.

Slow Cooked Beef Bourguignon

Tip:

Beef bourguignon is rich, hearty, and extra tender.

Course Main Course

Prep Time 20 minutes

Cook Time 9 hours 30 minutes

Ingredients

- Salt and pepper (to taste)
- 3 medium onions (diced)
- ¼ cup of tomato paste
- 6 medium garlic cloves minced (about 2 tablespoons minced garlic)
- ¼ cup of flour
- 1 cup of Kettle and Fire Chicken Bone Broth
- 2 bay leaves
- 10 ounces cremini mushrooms (or better still baby bella mushrooms roughly sliced)
- Chopped parsley (for garnishing)
- 1 (about 5-pound) boneless beef chuck eye roast
- 8 ounces (about 6 slices) bacon cut into ¼ -inch pieces
- 1 medium carrot (peeled and finely chopped)

2 teaspoons of brown sugar

1 tablespoon of fresh thyme leaves minced (or better still 1 teaspoon dried thyme)

1 (about 750-ml) bottle pinot noir or better still any medium-bodied red wine

1/3 cup of soy sauce

2 cups of frozen pearl onions

1 cup of sweet peas

Directions:

1. First, trim beef chuck eye roast and cut into 1 ½ -inch pieces.
2. After which you place the prepared beef in a 6-quart slow cooker and season with salt and pepper.
3. After that, cook bacon for about 8 minutes in a large nonstick skillet over medium heat until crisp.
4. At this point, you transfer the bacon to a plate lined with paper towels, leaving the fat in the skillet (NOTE: refrigerate the bacon until serving time).
5. This is when you pour off all but 2 tablespoons of the bacon fat in the skillet.
6. Then you add carrot, sugar, thyme, onions, tomato paste, garlic, and a pinch of salt.
7. Furthermore, cook for about 10-12 minutes over medium-high heat until the vegetables are softened and lightly browned.
8. After which you sprinkle flour all over the vegetables, stirring to coat.
9. Then stir in wine, scraping up any browned bits, bring to a simmer, and cook to allow the alcohol evaporates, 10-12 minutes.
10. In addition, pour the mixture over the beef in the slow cooker.

11. Stir in chicken bone broth, soy sauce and bay leaves until evenly combined, then cover and cook on low for 9-11 hours or on high for 5-7 hours, until meat is tender.
12. At about 30 minutes before serving, add frozen pearl onions, mushrooms, and sweet peas in the slow cooker (NOTE: cook on low until the pearl onions and mushrooms are cooked through).
13. At this point, when the cooking is done, let the cooking liquid settle for 5 minutes, then remove as much fat as possible from the surface using a large spoon.
14. Remove the bay leaves, taste and season with salt and pepper if desired.
15. After that, reheat the bacon in a microwave on high power for 30 seconds.
16. Make sure you serve the beef burgundy over mashed potatoes and sprinkle individual portions with the bacon.
17. Finally, garnish with chopped parsley.

Recipe Notes

1. Remember, if you want to make this recipe gluten-free, I suggest you substitute Tamari or coconut aminos for the soy sauce and replace the flour with 3 tablespoons cornstarch as a thickening agent.
2. If you using cornstarch, I suggest you dissolve it in 1/3 cup cold water, then add the mixture at step 4 after the wine is evaporated.

Salsa de Guajillo

Prep Time 10 minutes

Total Time 10 minutes

Servings 3 cups

Ingredients

    1/3 cup of white onion (sliced)

    ½ cup of Kettle and Fire Chicken Bone Broth

    ½ teaspoon of salt

    4 Roma tomatoes (toasted)

    1 small clove garlic

    6 guajillo chilies (toasted)

Directions:

1. Meanwhile, heat oven to 350°F.
2. After which you toast Roma tomatoes and guajillo chilies together for 10 minutes.
3. After that, you flip the chilies halfway through the toasting time.
4. Then place all prepared ingredients in a food processor or blender and blend well.
5. Finally, use a colander to filter out any solid pieces to ensure a smooth salsa if you like. (I usually skip this step.)

Chicken Mushroom Risotto

Tips:

This recipe makes a savory, rich, and velvety chicken risotto in seven simple steps, totally gluten free and ready in forty minutes.

Course Main Course

Prep Time 10 minutes

Cook Time 30 minutes

Servings 4

Ingredients

- 2 garlic cloves (minced)
- ½ cup of carrots (diced)
- 1 cup of Arborio rice
- ½ teaspoon of dried thyme
- 6 ounces' mushrooms (sliced)
- 1 cup of shredded chicken (cooked)
- Freshly ground black pepper
- 3 tablespoons of olive oil
- 1 small onion (diced)
- Sea salt (to taste)
- ½ cup of white wine (it is optional)
- 3 cups of Kettle and Fire Mushroom Chicken Bone Broth
- 8 ounces frozen Brussels sprouts
- ¼ cup of chopped fresh parsley

½ cup of freshly grated parmesan cheese

Directions:

1. First, you heat olive oil over medium heat in a medium saucepan.
2. After which you add garlic and cook until fragrant.
3. After that, place onion and carrots in the saucepan, add a pinch of salt, and turn the heat up to high.
4. Then cook until the onions are translucent, stirring often, about 1 minute.
5. At this point, stir in rice, followed by thyme (NOTE: let the rice toast in the saucepan and coat with oil until it starts turning slightly brown, stirring often, about 2-3 minutes).
6. This is when you add wine and continue stirring until the alcohol evaporates, about 1 minute.
7. Furthermore, pour chicken broth into the pan and bring to a boil.
8. Then, once it's boiling, stir in mushrooms and Brussels sprouts and bring to a boil again, stirring occasionally.
9. After which you add shredded chicken and turn the heat down to low.
10. Cover and simmer for about 15 minutes until the chicken broth is absorbed by the rice.
11. In addition, uncover, stir in parsley and Parmesan cheese.
12. Make sure you keep stirring until the cheese is melted; turn off the heat.
13. After that, season with freshly ground black pepper.
14. Finally, transfer the risotto to serving bowls and garnish with more parsley.
15. Serve immediately.

Recipe Notes

Feel free to substitute wine for more bone broth.

Easy New Orleans Slow Cooker Shrimp Jambalaya

Tip:

This recipe is spicy, hearty, and protein-packed.

Course Main Course

Prep Time 20 minutes

Cook Time 3 hours

Servings 6

Ingredients

- 6 ounces Andouille sausage (or better still any type of smoked sausage) sliced
- 1 medium red onion (chopped)
- 8 ounces' white mushrooms (sliced)
- 4 cloves of garlic pressed (or better still minced)
- 2 ½ cups of Kettle and Fire Chicken Bone Broth
- 1 tablespoon of olive oil
- ½ teaspoon of sea salt
- ½ teaspoon of thyme
- 1 teaspoon of ground cumin
- 2 cups of jasmine rice (or regular white rice)
- 12 ounces of boneless skinless chicken breasts (finely diced)
- 1 green bell pepper (finely diced)
- 2 celery stalks (chopped)
- 2 cups of tomato (diced)

1 tablespoon of cilantro leaves (finely chopped)

1/3 cup of tomato paste

1 teaspoon of Louisiana hot sauce

½ teaspoon of cayenne pepper

½ teaspoon of ground pepper

12 ounces' raw large shrimp (peeled and deveined)

Directions:

1. First, you place all the ingredients in your crockpot, excluding shrimp and rice; stir well.
2. After which you set the crockpot on high and cook for about 2-3 hours.
3. Then, about 40 minutes before serving, add rice and shrimp to the crockpot.
4. At this point, stir and make sure the rice is completely covered.
5. Finally, you continue cooking on high for 40 minutes, until the rice is tender.

Recipe Notes

1. If using brown rice, I suggest you prepare to stir it into the crock pot an hour before serving, because brown rice takes more time to cook.
2. I recommend enjoying this jambalaya the same day as it's cooked, if you want to get the best results.
3. Remember, storing any leftovers will likely affect the rice texture.
4. Nevertheless, you can totally cook the rice separately and pour the crock pot jambalaya mixture over the cooked rice; enjoy the leftovers as well!

Healthy Greek Quinoa Salad with Simple Lemon Dressing

Tip:

This recipe is healthy and delicious.

Course Salad

Prep Time 5 minutes

Cook Time 20 minutes

Servings 8

Ingredients

- 3 ½ cups of Kettle and Fire Chicken Bone Broth
- 1-pint cherry tomatoes (halved)
- Kosher salt (to taste)
- Juice of 1 lemon
- 2 cups of uncooked quinoa
- 1 (5-ounce) package spring mix
- ¼ cup of extra-virgin olive oil
- Freshly ground black pepper (to taste)

Directions:

1. First, rinse quinoa under cold running water.
2. After which you transfer cleaned quinoa to a large saucepan, add bone broth, and bring to a boil.
3. After that, switch heat to low and let it simmer for about 15-25 minutes, until the quinoa is tender and all the liquid has been absorbed.

4. Then, once the quinoa is cooked, remove from heat and let cool completely.
5. Furthermore, in a large bowl or in the same saucepan, add cherry tomatoes, pepper, spring mix, olive oil, salt, and lemon juice.
6. Finally, mix until all ingredients are well combined.

Slow Cooker Curry Chicken

Tip:

This recipe is made with juicy chicken thighs in a mild curry sauce, then slow-cooked with spices, fresh veggies, and coconut milk.

Course Main Course

Prep Time 20 minutes

Cook Time 4 hours

Servings 8

Ingredients

- ¼ cup of cornstarch
- 4 pounds of bone-in chicken thighs skin removed and fat trimmed
- Salt and pepper

INGREDIENTS FOR THE CURRY SAUCE:

- 3 tablespoons of mild or sweet curry powder
- 1 tablespoon of turmeric
- 1 jalapeño pepper (seeded and minced)
- 1 tablespoon of fresh ginger (minced)
- Salt (to taste)
- 3 tablespoons of soy sauce (**NOTE:** substitute coconut aminos for a gluten-free version of this recipe)
- 3 tablespoons of coconut oil
- 1 teaspoon of garam masala

2 medium white onions (chopped)

4 cloves garlic (minced)

2 tablespoons of tomato paste

2 ½ cups of Kettle and Fire Chicken Bone Broth

INGREDIENTS FOR THE SLOW COOKER:

4 medium carrots scrubbed and cut into 1-inch pieces

2 Roma tomatoes (chopped)

¼ cup of fresh cilantro

1 ½ pounds red potatoes scrubbed and cut into 1-inch pieces

1 cup of frozen peas

1 cup of coconut milk

Directions:

1. First, season chicken with salt and pepper and coat with cornstarch; set aside.
2. After which you heat coconut oil in a large skillet over medium heat until shimmering.
3. After that, add curry powder, garam masala, and turmeric and cook for about 10 seconds until fragrant.
4. Then, stir in onions, garlic, jalapeño pepper, ginger, tomato paste and a pinch of salt and cook, stirring often, until the onions are lightly browned and softened, about 10 minutes.
5. At this point, add chicken broth into the skillet, scraping up any browned bits.
6. This is when you add soy sauce or coconut aminos; stir well.
7. Furthermore, you cook until slightly thickened; remove from heat.

8. After which you place potatoes and carrots in a 6-quart slow cooker, followed by the chicken.
9. Then, pour the curry sauce over the chicken and cover.
10. Cook on low for 4-5 hours or until the chicken is tender.
11. This is when you let the cooking liquid settle for 5 minutes and remove fat from the surface using a big spoon.
12. In addition, stir in tomatoes, peas, coconut milk and cilantro.
13. Finally, let it stand until the peas and tomatoes are heated through, about 5 minutes or longer.
14. Make sure you taste, season with salt and pepper if desired before serving.

Creamy Mushroom Pasta

Tip:

This recipe is an easy and decadent weekday meal you can look forward to, ready in 20 minutes and requires only 10 basic ingredients.

Course Main Course

Prep Time 5 minutes

Cook Time 15 minutes

Servings 6

Ingredients

- 1 tablespoon of unsalted butter
- 8 ounces' white button mushrooms (stems removed)
- ¼ cup of heavy cream
- Salt (to taste)
- Chopped fresh parsley (for garnishing)
- 1 serving pasta (I prefer whole wheat linguine.)
- 2 garlic cloves (minced)
- 2 tablespoons of dry white wine
- ¼ cup of Kettle and Fire Chicken Bone Broth
- ¼ cup of grated parmesan cheese
- Freshly ground black pepper

Directions:

1. First, in a large pot, cook pasta in salted boiling water for 8-9 minutes according to the package directions or until al dente; drain.
2. In the meantime, in a large skillet, melt butter over medium-high heat.
3. After which you stir in minced garlic and let it cook for about 30 seconds until fragrant.
4. After that, place mushrooms in the skillet, cut side up.
5. Then cook for 3-5 minutes or until mushrooms start shrinking, moving them around with a spatula occasionally.
6. Furthermore, add white wine; continue cooking to let the wine and mushroom juice evaporate, about 3 minutes.
7. At this point, pour heavy cream and chicken bone broth into the skillet, add a generous pinch of salt.
8. This is when you switch to medium heat and cook until the cooking liquid is slightly thickened, flipping the mushrooms a couple times.
9. In addition, spread parmesan cheese over the mushrooms and gently stir until the cheese is melted (NOTE: taste and add more salt if desired).
10. After which you toss the cooked pasta into the skillet.
11. After that, combine well with the mushroom mixture, then transfer to a serving plate.
12. Then, sprinkle with freshly ground black pepper and garnish with chopped parsley.
13. Finally, add more grated parmesan cheese if desired. Enjoy!

Recipe Notes

I prefer whole white button mushrooms (NOTE: feel free to use sliced Portobello mushrooms or baby bella mushrooms for this recipe).

To make more servings, I will suggest you double the ingredients.

Southern Collard Greens with Bone Broth

Tip:

This recipe is juicy, flavorful, and delicious; cooked to tender perfection with bone broth, southern-style comfort food just got healthier.

Course Main Course, Side Dish

Prep Time 10 minutes

Cook Time 55 minutes

Servings 8

Ingredients

- 1 medium sweet onion (diced)
- 3 garlic cloves (minced)
- Freshly ground black pepper
- 4 slices bacon (cut into ¼ -inch pieces)
- Kosher salt
- 3 cups of Kettle and Fire Chicken Bone Broth
- 6 bunches fresh collard greens stemmed and roughly chopped (about 2 pounds)

Directions:

1. First, adjust an oven rack to lower-middle position and heat the oven to 350°F.

2. After which you cook bacon in a large Dutch oven over medium-high heat for about 2 minutes until the fat starts to render.
3. After that, stir in onions and a pinch of salt.
4. At this point, cook until the onions are softened, about 5-7 minutes.
5. Then add garlic and stir for 30 seconds.
6. Furthermore, add bone broth and bring to a simmer.
7. After which you add the greens, a handful at a time, until wilted.
8. Then cover and place the pot in the oven; cook for 45 minutes or until the greens are tender.
9. Finally, remove from oven; season with more salt and black pepper.
10. Make sure you serve with hot sauce.

Recipe Notes

a. Remember that the leftover cooking liquid can be used to cook another batch of collard greens. Or better still dip your cornbread or biscuit in the flavorful cooking liquid.
b. If you don't have a Dutch oven, I suggest you use a heavy-duty roasting pan that is stovetop safe and follow the instructions. When ready to bake, make sure you cover with aluminum foil.

Turkey Pot Pie

Tip:

This recipe is perfect for a rainy day.

Course Main Course

Prep Time 10 minutes

Cook Time 50 minutes

Servings 6

Ingredients

- 1 cup of potatoes (diced)
- 1 cup of celery (diced)
- Salt and pepper (to taste)
- ½ cup of all-purpose flour
- 1 cup of milk
- 1 pie crust
- 3 tablespoons of butter
- 1 cup onions (diced)
- 1 cup of carrots (diced)
- 1 tablespoon of fresh thyme leaves minced (or better still 1 teaspoon dried thyme)
- 1 cup of Kettle and Fire Chicken Bone Broth
- 2 cups of turkey (cooked and chopped)

Directions:

1. Meanwhile, heat oven to 400°F.

2. After which in a large non-stick skillet, melt butter over medium-high heat.
3. After that, add onions, celery, potatoes, and carrots in the skillet.
4. Then, add a pinch of salt and pepper to taste.
5. At this point, sauté for about 10 minutes or until the vegetables are tender.
6. Then you stir in thyme leaves while cooking.
7. Furthermore, sprinkle flour into the pan; cook for one more minute, stirring constantly.
8. This is when you gradually stir in broth and milk.
9. After which you reduce heat to medium and cook until the mixture is thickened and bubbly, stirring constantly.
10. Then, add turkey and stir well.
11. In addition, pour the mixture into a 9-inch pie dish and top with pie crust.
12. After that, trim off the excess crust alongside the edge of your pie dish; cut slits in the middle to allow steam to escape.
13. Finally, bake the pie for about 40-50 minutes or until pastry is golden brown and the filling is bubbly and cooked through.

Slow Cooker Split Pea Soup

Tip:

This recipe is loaded with vegetables, fiber, and flavor; only 10 minutes of prep time, fewer than ten ingredients, and its gluten-free.

Course Soup

Prep Time 10 minutes

Cook Time 8 hours

Servings 8

Ingredients

- 2 cloves garlic (minced)
- 1 ½ teaspoons of kosher salt
- 2 cups carrots (diced)
- 1 cup of celery (diced)
- Cooked bacon pieces for serving and chopped cilantro for garnishing
- 1 cup of yellow onions (diced)
- ½ teaspoon of dried oregano
- 1 teaspoon of ground black pepper
- 1 cup of red potatoes (diced)
- 1 pound dried split peas
- 8 cups Kettle and Fire Beef Bone Broth (4 cartons)

Directions:

1. First, place all ingredients in a 4-quart (or bigger) slow cooker.
2. After which you cover and cook on low for 8-10 hours.
3. After that, taste to adjust the flavor by adding more salt if desired.
4. Finally, ladle into serving bowls and top with cooked bacon pieces and fresh cilantro leaves before serving. Enjoy!

French Onion Soup

Course Soup

Prep Time 10 minutes

Cook Time 20 hours 22 minutes

Servings 12

Ingredients

- 2 tablespoons of butter unsalted
- 1 teaspoon of salt (plus more to taste)
- 2 tablespoons of balsamic vinegar
- 3 tablespoons of Sherry (optional)
- 3 pounds of yellow onions (peeled and sliced)
- 2 tablespoons of olive oil
- Freshly ground black pepper
- 10 cups of Kettle and Fire Beef Bone Broth

Ingredients for assembling the soup:

- Chopped parsley for garnishing
- 6 baguette slices for each bowl
- 1/3-2 cups of grated or better still shaved Gruyere cheese

Directions:

1. First, place onions in a 6-quart slow cooker.
2. After which you stir in butter and olive oil.

3. After that, season with salt and pepper; cover and cook on low for 12 hours.
4. Then, add balsamic vinegar and beef bone broth into the slow cooker (add sherry if using).
5. At this point, you cover and cook on low for another 6-8 hours.
6. Meanwhile, heat oven to 350°F.
7. Furthermore, portion and ladle the soup and onions into oven-safe bowls and place the bowls on a baking sheet.
8. After that, top each bowl with a slice of toast and a generous amount of grated or shaved Gruyere cheese.
9. This is when you bake on a rack in the upper third of the oven for 20-30 minutes or until the cheese is melted.
10. In addition, switch oven to broil and broil the soup for about 2-3 minutes until the cheese is browned.
11. Finally, garnish with chopped parsley and serve warm.

Cream of Chicken Soup Recipe

Tip:

This homemade cream of chicken soup is better tasting and requires only 4 ingredients; ready in 15 minutes.

Course Soup

Prep Time 2 minutes

Cook Time 13 minutes

Servings 3 cups

Ingredients

- 1/2 cup of all-purpose flour
- 2 cups of Kettle and Fire Chicken Bone Broth (1 carton)
- 2 cups of organic milk (use low-fat if you prefer)

Ingredients for the seasoning

- ½ teaspoon of garlic
- ½ teaspoon of dried parsley
- ½ teaspoon of onion powder
- ½ teaspoon of ground black pepper
- 1 teaspoon of sea salt

Directions:

1. First, in a medium saucepan, bring chicken bone broth to a boil over medium-high heat.

2. After which in a separate medium mixing bowl, whisk together milk and flour until the flour is dissolved.
3. After that, slowly add milk and flour mixture into the boiling broth, whisking constantly to combine.
4. Then you reduce heat to medium; add all seasonings and bring the mixture to a slow boil, continuously whisking.
5. At this point, let the mixture boil for about 3 minutes or until thickened.
6. Finally, use in a recipe immediately or store in an airtight jar and refrigerate for up to a week.

Recipe Notes

1. Feel free to play with the seasonings.
2. If you'd like your cream of chicken soup thicker, I suggest you add more flour. Remember, the soup will thicken even more after cooled.

White Bean Chili

Tip:

This hearty and healthy recipe takes only five steps and 25 minutes; it is also a perfect way to use up your leftovers for a nourishing weekday meal.

Course Main Course

Prep Time 10 minutes

Cook Time 25 minutes

Servings 4

Ingredients

- 1 medium onion (chopped)
- 1 (about 4-oz) can chopped green chili peppers
- 2 teaspoons of ground cumin
- 4 cups of Kettle and Fire Chicken Bone Broth (2 cartons)
- 2 (about 15-oz) cans white beans (great northern, cannellini or chickpea)
- Fresh parsley leaves (for garnishing)
- 1 tablespoon of coconut oil
- 3 cloves garlic (crushed)
- 8 ounces' mushrooms (sliced)
- 1 teaspoon of dried oregano
- 4 cups of cooked turkey (diced)
- 1 cup of shredded Monterey Jack cheese

Directions:

1. First, heat the oil in a large saucepan over medium heat.
2. After which you add onion and garlic; Slowly cook until fragrant.
3. After that, mix in the green chili peppers, cumin, mushroom and oregano.
4. At this point, continue to cook and stir the mixture until tender, about 3 minutes.
5. This is when you add bone broth, turkey, and white beans.
6. Furthermore, simmer 15 minutes, stirring occasionally.
7. Finally, dish the chili; add cheese and garnish with parsley leaves. Enjoy!

Recipe Notes

You can make this recipe with cooked chicken.

Chicken Tortilla Soup

Course Soup

Prep Time 15 minutes

Cook Time 30 minutes

Servings 6

Ingredients

- 2 cups of frozen carrots and peas
- 2 cups of shredded chicken
- 2 cups of zucchini (diced)
- ½ cup of white onion (diced)
- 1/8 teaspoon Ghost Pepper Hot Sauce or better still your desired hot sauce (optional)

Ingredients for the soup base:

- ½ cup of white onion (roughly sliced)
- 3 large cloves garlic
- salt (to taste)
- 8-10 Roma tomatoes or better still 1 (32-oz) can diced tomatoes
- 1 cup of cilantro firmly packed
- 2 cups of Kettle and Fire Chicken Bone Broth 1 carton

Ingredients for the topping:

- 2 cups of tortilla chips crushed and divided (Use corn chips for a gluten-free version)

2 avocados (sliced and divided)

1 cup of shredded cheddar cheese (divided)

Fresh cilantro (for garnishing)

Lime or lemon wedges (for serving)

DIRECTIONS:

1. Meanwhile, heat oven to 350°F.
2. After which you roast Roma tomatoes for 10 minutes.
3. Meanwhile, chop up vegetables.
4. Then, when tomatoes are done, allow to cool.
5. At this point, quarter each one and place into your food processor or blender with garlic, roughly sliced onion, cilantro.
6. After that, add chicken broth and a pinch of salt; blend until smooth. (NOTE: Depending on the size of your blender, you might need to process two or three batches to finish up the ingredients)
7. This is when you pour soup base into a saucepan and bring to a boil.
8. Furthermore, in a sauté pan, melt butter and sauté diced onion over high heat until fragrant.
9. Add carrots and cook for 5 minutes; add diced zucchini into the pan.
10. Then cook until the vegetables are tender.
11. In addition, transfer cooked vegetables into the soup base.
12. After which you add sweet peas and bring to a boil again; stir in shredded chicken.
13. After that, reduce to medium heat and simmer for 15 minutes; stir occasionally.
14. Then, taste and adjust the flavor by adding more salt if desired.

15. At this point, drop in hot sauce; stir until even (this is optional).
16. Finally, Dish; Top with tortilla chips, cheddar cheese, avocado slices, cilantro for each serving.
17. You can squeeze a dash of fresh lime juice. Enjoy!

Salsa Verde Recipe

Course sauce

Prep Time 10 minutes

Total Time 10 minutes

Servings 3 cups

Ingredients

- 2 avocados
- ½ teaspoon of salt
- 1 cup of Kettle and Fire Chicken Bone Broth
- 8 oz. tomatillos
- 5 serrano peppers
- 1/3 cup of white onion (sliced)
- ½ cup of cilantro loosely packed

Directions:

1. First, place all prepared ingredients in a food processor or blender.
2. Then, blend well and preserve.

Recipe Notes

Remember to put one of the avocado seeds in the salsa when preserving to prevent color from changing.

Red White and Blue Kansas-City Style BBQ Bone Broth

Ingredients:

A dash of allspice

A dash of paprika

1 pat of grass-fed butter

1 tablespoon of apple cider vinegar

A dash of chili powder

1 teaspoon of ketchup

1 teaspoon of coconut aminos

Directions:

1. First, combine all ingredients with 8 oz. bone broth and heat to a boil.
2. After which you reduce to low and simmer for 5-15 minutes.
3. Enjoy warm.

Veggie-Packed Dairy-Free Creamy Broccoli Soup

Tip:

This recipe combines the magic of nostalgic comfort food with a paleo, veggie-based set of ingredients that will leave you feeling full and satisfied.

Prep Time 10 minutes

Cook Time 15 minutes

Servings 8

Ingredients

- 2 cloves garlic minced (or better still ½ teaspoon garlic powder)
- 3 cups of coarsely chopped sun chokes Jerusalem artichokes
- 3 cups of Kettle and Fire chicken bone broth plus more for cooking
- 1 teaspoon of sea salt
- Salt and black pepper (to taste)
- 1 large onion (chopped)
- 3 tablespoons of extra virgin olive oil plus more for cooking and garnish
- 1 small head fresh cauliflower about 6 cups cauliflower stems and florets (chopped coarsely)
- 1 head fresh broccoli about 5 cups broccoli stems and florets (chopped coarsely)
- 1 teaspoon of apple cider vinegar

Optional Topping:

Fresh scallions (chopped)

Directions:

1. First, heat a large pot over medium heat.
2. After which you add olive oil, onions, and garlic.
3. After that, sauté until translucent (about 3 minutes); add sun chokes and cauliflower, stirring to coat, and sauté for another 3 to 5 minutes.
4. Then, add 3 cups chicken broth and turn up to medium-high heat and cover.
5. At this point, cook for 10 minutes or until the sun chokes are fork tender; while that's cooking, heat a skillet to medium heat and add another teaspoon of olive oil.
6. This is when you add broccoli florets and salt, sautéing for about 5 minutes, then add a few splashes of bone broth to soften the broccoli a bit further.
7. Furthermore, once the sun chokes and cauliflower are well-cooked and soft, either use an immersion blender or transfer to a regular blender to completely blend the mixture; return to the pot after blended.
8. After which you turn heat down to low and add coconut milk, apple cider vinegar, and black pepper.
9. In additionally, stir to incorporate; stir in broccoli and cover for another 2–3 minutes.
10. Finally, op with fresh scallions and a drizzle of olive oil, and serve piping hot.

Slow Cooker Chicken Bone Broth Recipe

Tip:

This recipe is a Kettle & Fire tested that features organic chicken bones, fresh vegetables, and herbs.

Course Bone Broth

Prep Time 15 minutes

Cook Time 12 hours

Servings 16 cups

Ingredients

- 2 stalks celery (roughly chopped)
- 1 yellow or white onion (roughly chopped)
- 1 head garlic
- ¼ cup of fresh thyme
- 2 bay leaves
- 8-10 cups of filtered water (or better still enough to cover ingredients)
- 2 pounds of chicken bones leftover from roasted chicken, preferably organic
- 2 carrots skin on (roughly chopped)
- 1 green bell pepper (roughly chopped)
- ½ cup of fresh parsley
- 2 sprigs of rosemary
- 1 tablespoon of whole peppercorns

Directions:

1. First, rinse vegetables and herbs and place into a slow cooker.
2. After which you add chicken bones and all remaining ingredients to slow cooker and cover with enough water so that all ingredients are submerged.
3. After that, turn on slow cooker to low heat and let cook for about 12-18 hours.
4. Then, remove from heat and carefully separate the vegetables and bones from the broth.
5. At this point, strain the broth into a bowl through a colander, and strain once more through a cheesecloth to remove any remaining particles.
6. Finally, pour broth into an airtight jar and store in the refrigerator for up to a week, or freeze for up to 3 months.

Bone Broth Gazpacho Recipe with Cilantro Chimichurri

Tip:

This recipe is a refreshing way to serve up summer vegetables and rich bone broth!

Course Soup

Prep Time 15 minutes

Cook Time 30 minutes

Servings 4

Ingredients

- 2 large bell peppers
- ½ medium beet
- ¼ cup of olive oil
- Sea salt and pepper (to taste)
- 2 large tomatoes
- ¼ habanero pepper (deseeded)
- 1 ½ cups of Kettle and Fire Chicken Bone Broth
- 2 tablespoons of balsamic vinegar

Ingredients for the Cilantro Chimichurri:

- 1 clove garlic
- ¼ cup of extra virgin olive oil
- Salt and pepper (to taste)

1 cup of packed cilantro

1 teaspoon diced jalapeño (deseeded)

½ lime

Ingredients for garnish:

Fresh cilantro leaves

Salt and pepper (to taste)

Freshly cooked corn

Directions:

1. Meanwhile, heat the oven to 400°F.
2. After which you bring a small saucepan of water to a boil.
3. After that, roughly chop tomatoes, bell peppers, and carefully deseeded habanero.
4. Then, drizzle with 1 tablespoon olive oil, and spread on sheet pan.
5. At this point, roast for about 20-25 minutes, or until slightly charred and tender.
6. In the meanwhile, boil 1 small beet for about 20 minutes, or until tender when poked with fork; remove and let cool.
7. Furthermore, in a food processor, combine all ingredients for chimichurri; pulse until well combined.
8. When tomatoes and peppers are ready, add all gazpacho ingredients to a high-speed blender and blend on high for 50-60 seconds, or until completely smooth.
9. In addition, chill in refrigerator for at least 1-2 hours, or store in airtight container for up to 5 days before consuming.

10. Finally, pour into bowls and garnish with fresh corn and cilantro chimichurri. Enjoy!

Recipe Notes

Remember that the habanero gives the gazpacho a bit of a fiery kick, so if you'd prefer a milder option, I suggest you skip the peppers.

COLLAGEN GLUTEN FREE RECIPES

Creamy Tomato Soup with Coconut and Curry

TIP:

This creamy tomato soup is a wholesome, dairy-free version of the classic that's sure to become one of your new favorite homemade tomato soup recipes.

Course Soup

Prep Time 5 minutes

Cook Time 40 minutes

Servings 4

Ingredients

- 1 red onion (chopped)
- 1 carrot (chopped)
- 1 clove garlic (minced)
- 2 teaspoons of curry powder
- 1 cup of canned full-fat coconut milk
- Freshly ground black pepper
- 2 tablespoons of coconut oil
- 1 red bell pepper (chopped)
- Kosher salt
- 24 ounces canned whole peeled tomatoes
- 1 ½ cups Kettle and Fire Chicken Bone Broth
- 1 lime (cut into quarters)

Optional garnish: Microgreens and hemp seeds

Directions:

1. First, in a medium pot over medium-high heat, warm the coconut oil until melted.
2. After which you add the onion, bell pepper, carrot, and a pinch of salt and cook, stirring occasionally, for 4 to 6 minutes until the vegetables are soft.
3. After that, add the garlic and curry powder and cook until fragrant, about 1 minute.
4. At this point, stir in the tomatoes and a pinch of salt; cook, stirring, for another minute.
5. This is when you add the broth and simmer until the tomatoes are cooked, 10 to 15 minutes.
6. Furthermore, remove from the heat and blend until smooth with an immersion blender or regular blender.
7. After that, return to the stove over medium heat.
8. In addition, stir in the coconut milk and a squeeze of lime and cook for another minute.
9. Finally, season with salt and pepper to taste.
10. Then, garnish with microgreens and hemp seeds, if using.

Creamy Potato Leek Soup

Course Main Course, Soup

Prep Time 15 minutes

Cook Time 45 minutes

Servings 6

Ingredients

- 2 tablespoons of avocado oil (divided) or better still olive oil, plus more for green leek topper
- 10 fingerling potatoes (cut into 1-inch pieces)
- 6 cups of Kettle and Fire Beef Bone Broth
- 2 bay leaves
- 2 teaspoons of apple cider vinegar
- 2 large leeks white and green parts separated and chopped into ¼ inch pieces
- 4 medium celery roots or better still 2 large ones (peeled and cubed)
- ½ large cauliflower or 1 small one, large cored and chunked into 2-inch pieces
- 2 cups of water
- 3 teaspoons of salt
- **OPTIONAL:** 6 strips of uncured bacon (broiled and crumbled)
- **OPTIONAL:** freshly ground black pepper

Directions:

1. First, in a large stockpot over medium heat, warm 1 tablespoon avocado oil.
2. After which you add white part of leeks and cook until they become translucent.
3. After that, add potatoes, broth, water, celery root, cauliflower, and bay leaves to the pot.
4. At this point, cover, increase to high heat and bring to a boil; then lower to medium heat.
5. Furthermore, cook until potatoes are soft, about 40 minutes; while the soup is cooking, heat the oven to 400°F.
6. After which you toss the green part of the leeks, 1 tablespoon avocado oil, and a generous pinch of salt.
7. This is when you lay out flat on a large sheet pan and roast for 10 minutes, or until just browned; set aside.
8. In addition, remove the bay leaves from the soup and discard.
9. After that, turn heat to low and transfer all of the cauliflower and half of the other ingredients into a high-speed blender; blend until smooth.
10. Then stir blended contents into the rest of the ingredients; stir in apple cider vinegar.
11. Finally, ladle into bowls and top with green leek tops, crumbled bacon and black pepper (if using).
12. Make sure you serve piping hot.

Creamy Asparagus Soup with Avocado and Fennel

Course Soup

Prep Time 5 minutes

Cook Time 40 minutes

Servings 4

Ingredients

- 1 large leek white and pale green parts (finely chopped)
- Kosher salt
- 2 pounds of asparagus trimmed and cut into 1-inch pieces
- 1 lemon juiced
- Greek yogurt for serving (it is optional)
- 2 tablespoons of olive oil + more for serving
- 1 bulb fennel (thinly sliced)
- 4 cups of Kettle and Fire Chicken Bone Broth
- 1 tablespoon of lemon thyme leaves (minced)
- 1 avocado (peeled, pitted, and diced)
- Freshly ground black pepper

Directions:

1. First, in a large saucepan over medium-low heat, warm oil; add leek and fennel and a large pinch of salt.
2. After which you cook, stirring frequently, until fully softened but not browned, 3 to 5 minutes.

3. After that, stir in bone broth and bring to a simmer.
4. Add asparagus and thyme; bring to a simmer and cook for 1 minute.
5. Then, remove a few asparagus tips and use them for garnish.
6. Furthermore, continue simmering soup until asparagus is soft, 4 to 5 minutes.
7. At this point, remove from heat and add lemon juice and avocado.
8. This is when you blend soup using an immersion blender or in batches using a blender until it's smooth.
9. Finally, season to taste with salt and pepper and serve.
10. Make sure you garnish with reserved asparagus tips, fennel fronds, olive oil and Greek yogurt, if using.

Black Bean Soup with Smoked Paprika and Chipotle

Tip: this recipe is Smoky, smooth, and just a bit spicy, reinvents the American classic with a little Southwestern kick.

Course Main Course, Soup

Prep Time 10 minutes

Cook Time 25 minutes

Servings 4

Ingredients

- 1 onion (chopped)
- 2 garlic cloves (minced)
- 1 teaspoon of dried oregano
- 1 ¼ cup of cherry tomatoes halved (save some for garnish)
- 15 ounces of canned black beans (rinsed)
- 1 bunch fresh cilantro
- 1 lime juiced
- ¼ cup of Greek yogurt optional
- 2 tablespoons of olive oil
- 2 carrots (chopped)
- 1 teaspoon of ground cumin
- ½ teaspoon of smoked paprika
- 2 cups of Kettle and Fire Chicken Bone Broth

Kosher salt

1 chipotle Chile in adobo sauce

1 avocado (optional)

Directions:

1. First, in a large pot over medium heat, warm the oil.
2. After which you add carrots, onion, and garlic and cook, stirring occasionally, until the vegetables soften, 5 to 7 minutes.
3. After which you add the cumin, oregano, paprika and 1 cup of the tomatoes and stir to combine.
4. Then, cook until the spices are fragrant, about 1 minute.
5. At this point, add the bone broth, black beans, and 1 teaspoon salt.
6. This is when you increase to medium-high heat and bring to a boil.
7. Furthermore, reduce heat to a simmer and cook until the tomatoes are cooked through and the flavors have melded, 10 to 15 minutes.
8. Remove from heat; add the chipotle, cilantro, half the lime juice, and transfer soup to a blender.
9. After which you puree on high until smooth.
10. Then, add a splash of water to adjust thickness, if necessary.
11. Season with salt to taste; add more lime juice if needed.
12. Finally, serve and garnish with remaining avocado, tomatoes, or Greek yogurt, if using.

Paleo Butternut Squash Soup

Tip:

This recipe is a rich, creamy comfort food that's often loaded with milk or heavy cream and butter.

Course Soup

Prep Time 10 minutes

Cook Time 1 hour 40 minutes

Servings 6

Ingredients

- 2 tablespoons of ghee or better still coconut oil
- 2 cloves garlic (chopped)
- 2 cups of Kettle and Fire Chicken Bone Broth
- ¼ teaspoon of sumac
- ½ teaspoon of cinnamon
- 1 teaspoon of apple cider vinegar
- 1 large butternut squash
- ½ large yellow onion (chopped)
- 1.5- inch piece fresh ginger (chopped)
- 1 teaspoon of sea salt + more to taste
- ¼ teaspoon of red chili flake
- 1 cup of water

¾ cup of canned coconut milk

OPTIONAL TOPPING: freshly ground black pepper extra virgin olive oil, fresh sage, and avocado oil for frying

Directions:

1. First, place whole squash in a shallow baking pan and bake at 425°F for 1 hour 20 minutes, turning half-way through.
2. Then, when the squash is ready (NOTE: it will give when you press on the skin), remove from the oven and cut in half.
3. After which you scoop out the seeds, remove skin, and discard.
4. After that, cut the roasted squash into 2-inch cubes; while the squash is baking, loosely chop the yellow onion and garlic.
5. Furthermore, in a large stock pot over medium heat, melt the ghee.
6. At this point, add the onions and cook until translucent, about 5 minutes.
7. This is when you add the garlic and ginger, stirring to make sure the garlic doesn't burn; stir in the squash and cook until combined, 3 minutes.
8. In addition, stir in the salt, bone broth, sumac, red chili and cinnamon.
9. After which you cover and cook for another 10 minutes; remove from the heat.
10. After that, transfer the soup to a blender and blend until smooth. (Optionally, leave ½ of the soup unblended for a chunkier soup).
11. Then, return the blended soup to the pot.
12. Turn the heat to low, then stir in water, coconut milk, and apple cider vinegar; cook for another minute or two until warmed through.
13. Finally, add salt and black pepper, to taste. Serve.

Optional Topping:

1. First, in a separate frying pan, heat avocado oil.
2. After which you add 3 to 4 sage leaves per person to the oil and fry until crisp, taking care not to burn them.
3. Then, drizzle each serving of butternut soup with a good extra virgin olive oil and top with fried sage.

Slow Cooker Creamy Sweet Potato Soup with Coconut and Pistachios

Tip:

This recipe is creamy, quick and delicious!

Course Main Course, Soup

Prep Time 5 minutes

Cook Time 4 hours 30 minutes

Servings 4

Ingredients

- 1 yellow onion (chopped)
- 2 carrot sticks (chopped)
- 5 cups Kettle and Fire Chicken Bone Broth
- 1 teaspoon of ground black pepper
- ¼ cup of pistachio nuts (roughly chopped)
- 2 large sweet potatoes (roughly chopped)
- 2 stalks celery (chopped)
- 2 cloves garlic (minced)
- 1 teaspoon salt
- 1 ½ cups of coconut milk

Directions:

1. First, place all ingredients except the coconut milk in a large slow cooker or crockpot.

2. After which you cook on high heat for 4 hours; remove and let cool slightly.
3. Furthermore, using an immersion blender, puree the soup until smooth; then stir in the coconut milk. NOTE: don't reduce the heat.
4. Then, let cook for 30 more minutes.
5. Finally, serve and garnish with pistachio nuts.

Lentil Soup with Mushroom Chicken Bone Broth

Tip:

This recipe contains dietary fiber, B vitamins, and antioxidants; The olive oil rounds out the flavor, while a touch of lemon juice (or red wine vinegar, if you have it) brightens it all up.

Course Main Course

Prep Time 10 minutes

Cook Time 40 minutes

Servings 2 people

Ingredients

- 1 slice bacon (cut into ¼ inch pieces)
- 1 carrot (chopped)
- 2 cloves garlic (minced)
- ¼ teaspoon of red pepper flakes
- 12 ounces canned diced tomatoes
- Freshly ground black pepper
- ¼ cup of Greek yogurt (optional)
- 2 tablespoons of extra virgin olive oil
- 1 yellow onion (chopped)
- 1 stalk celery (chopped)
- Kosher salt
- ½ cup of green lentils
- 4 cups of Kettle and Fire Mushroom Chicken Bone Broth

1 lemon juiced

2 tablespoons of parsley leave (chopped)

Directions:

1. First, in a medium pot over medium heat, warm 1 tablespoon oil until shimmering.
2. After which you add the bacon and cook just until the fat starts to render, 3 to 5 minutes.
3. After that, add the carrots, onion, celery, and a pinch of salt and cook, stirring, until the vegetables become soft, 8 to 10 minutes.
4. At this point, add the garlic and red pepper flakes; cook until fragrant, 1 to 2 minutes.
5. This is when you stir in the lentils; add the crushed tomatoes and bone broth.
6. Then, bring the soup to a boil, reduce heat to a simmer.
7. Furthermore, Cook, covered, until the lentils are soft, 20 to 25 minutes.
8. After that, add the lemon juice.
9. In addition, remove from the heat and season with salt and pepper.
10. Finally, garnish with the parsley and Greek yogurt, if using.

COLLAGEN GUT-FRIENDLY RECIPES

Pesto Zucchini Pasta (Whole 30 Approved)

Tip:

This recipe is extremely easy to make; the combination of fresh basil, garlic, and tomatoes will bring Italy right into your kitchen.

Course Main Course

Prep Time 30 minutes

Cook Time 5 minutes

Servings 4 people

Ingredients

- 3 cups of fresh basil
- 3 cloves of garlic
- ½ teaspoon of salt
- 1 large tomato (diced)
- 3 large zucchini spiralized
- ¼ cup of pine nuts
- ½ cup of extra-virgin olive oil
- ½ teaspoon of pepper
- 1 tablespoon of coconut oil

Directions:

1. First, remove the water from the zucchini pasta by placing it on a paper towel.

2. After which you generously sprinkle sea salt over all of the zoodles and let sit for 20 minutes. (**NOTE:** This will pull the moisture out of the zoodles so they are not soggy).
3. Furthermore, while the zoodles sit, make the pesto.
4. Then, in a food processor, puree the pine nuts, olive oil, basil, garlic, salt, and pepper for 2 minutes, or until fully smooth.
5. In addition, using another paper towel, pat the zoodles dry.
6. After that, in a medium saucepan over medium heat, warm the coconut oil.
7. This is when you add the zoodles to the pan with ½ cup of pesto and diced tomato.
8. After which you cook, stirring occasionally, for 5 minutes, or until the zoodles are warm.
9. Finally, garnish with any leftover pine nuts and preserve the remaining pesto for later use.

Quinoa Buddha Breakfast Bowl

Tip:

This recipe turns savory to sweet, with the addition of banana, mint, berries, maple syrup, and warming notes of cinnamon and vanilla.

Course Breakfast

Prep Time 5 minutes

Servings 1

Ingredients

- 2 tablespoons of hemp hearts
- 1 teaspoon of cinnamon ground
- 1 leaf fresh mint for garnish (it is optional)
- ½ cup of unsweetened coconut (or better still almond milk)
- 1 teaspoon of pure maple syrup (optional for added sweetness)
- 1 cup of cooked quinoa warm or better still cold
- 1 teaspoon of pure vanilla extract
- 1 teaspoon of slivered almonds
- ¾ cup fresh (or preferably frozen berries)
    - ½ banana (sliced)

Directions:

1. First, combine all ingredients in bowl except mint, berries, and nut milk.
2. After which you pour nut milk over ingredients, garnish with mint and berries.

3. Enjoy!

Baked Almond-Crusted Cod with Sautéed Bok Choy and Bell Peppers

Course Main Course

Prep Time 10 minutes

Cook Time 10 minutes

Servings 4 people

Ingredients

- 2 sprigs parsley leaves (minced)
- ¼ cup of stone ground mustard
- sea salt
- 4 tablespoons of avocado oil
- 2 red bell peppers (thinly sliced)
- ½ cup of slivered almonds (roughly chopped)
- 2 sprigs rosemary leaves (minced)
- 2 sprigs oregano leaves (minced)
- 2 tablespoons of apple cider vinegar
- Freshly ground black pepper
- 1 ¼ pounds fresh Rock Cod filets (or better still your favorite white fish)
- 6 baby bok choy stems and leaves separated and coarsely chopped
- 1 lemon (sliced into wedges)

Directions:

1. First, heat oven to 350°F.
2. After which in a small bowl, mix half the herbs, apple cider vinegar, mustard, and a pinch of salt and pepper until all ingredients are fully incorporated.
3. After that, grease a 9 x 13-inch baking dish or pan with 1 tablespoon of avocado oil and place the fish on top.
4. Then, spread an even layer of the mustard mixture over the top of each fillet.
5. Furthermore, you evenly distribute slivered almonds on top of each fillet.
6. At this point, drizzle a thin layer of avocado oil and another pinch of salt over the almonds.
7. This is when you transfer to the oven and bake until the fish is flakey and opaque, about 10 minutes.
8. In addition, broil for 2 minutes to brown slightly; quickly remove from the oven.
9. After which in a large frying pan over medium-high heat, warm 2 tablespoons of avocado oil.
10. After that, add pepper and bok choy stems and cook, stirring, until softened, about 2 minutes.
11. Then, add the bok choy leaves and cook until wilted, about 1 minute.
12. This is when you remove from the heat and stir in a few generous pinches of salt and pepper.
13. Finally, plate in large bowls with the veggies on the bottom with the fish on top; spoon the juices from the baking dish over the fish.
14. Make sure you garnish with a slice of lemon and remaining fresh chopped herbs.

Bone Broth Ice Cubes

Tip:

This recipe is the perfect way to get your dose of protein and collagen on warm summer nights.

Course Bone Broth

Prep Time 4 hours

Servings 6 2-inch ice cubes

Ingredients

- 6 ounces Kettle and Fire Chicken Bone Broth
- ½ teaspoon of turmeric powder
- 6 ounces of Kettle and Fire Beef Bone Broth
- 1 sprig fresh rosemary (cut into small pieces)
- 1 sprig sage leaves (4 to 5 leaves)

Directions:

1. First, using a food safe silicone ice cube tray pour Kettle and Fire Beef Bone Broth into half of the ice cube tray. (NOTE: We used a 6-slot ice cube tray in this recipe that created 2-inch cubes.)
2. After which you pour Kettle and Fire Chicken Bone Broth into the remaining half of the ice cube tray.
3. After that, tuck rosemary, sage or a mix of both in a few bone broth ice cube slots with the bone broth.
4. Then, mix in a little bit turmeric powder into the rest of the ice cube slots with bone broth. NOTE: use more turmeric if desired.

5. At this point, place the ice cube tray in a freezer for about 4-24 hours or until completely solid.
6. Finally, enjoy with any iced beverage of your choice for added nutrients!

Coconut Vegetable Curry Over Quinoa

Tip:

This recipe is a nourishing, aromatic curry containing veggies, herbs, and spices is one of the easiest (and most delicious) ways to support a health-conscious lifestyle.

Course Main Course

Prep Time 10 minutes

Cook Time 45 minutes

Servings 2

Ingredients

- 1 clove garlic (minced)
- 1 green onion (finely chopped)
- 2 medium zucchini (chopped)
- 1 cup of full-fat canned coconut milk
- 1 pinch of sea salt
- ¾ cup of cooked quinoa
- 1 tablespoon of coconut oil
- 1-inch piece ginger
- ¾ cup of Kettle and Fire Beef Bone Broth
- 2 small sweet potatoes (peeled and cubed)
- 2 tablespoons of garam masala
- 1 pinch freshly ground black pepper

2 tablespoons of chopped parsley

Directions:

1. First, in a saucepan over medium heat, melt coconut oil.
2. After which you add garlic, ginger and green onion and cook for about 5 minutes until onion is soft and translucent.
3. After that, add bone broth, zucchini, and sweet potato to the pot with the onions.
4. Then you cook, stirring occasionally, until the vegetables are tender, about 25 minutes.
5. In the meantime, in a separate small saucepan over low heat, warm coconut milk and garam masala, salt, and pepper; Cook, stirring frequently, until fragrant, about 15 minutes.
6. At this point, add the spiced coconut milk to the pot with the vegetables; add parsley, and stir to combine.
7. This is when you turn the heat to low, cover, and simmer for about 10 minutes longer.
8. Furthermore, remove from heat and discard the piece of ginger.
9. In addition, place quinoa on a plate and top with curry.
10. Finally, garnish with extra parsley or cilantro and enjoy!

Sweet Potato Toast (Whole30 Approved)

Tips:

This is one of the easiest and most satisfying comfort food breakfasts you'll ever have.

This recipe calls for oven-roasted sweet potatoes, which makes it Whole30 Plan approved and paleo friendly.

Course Breakfast

Prep Time 5 minutes

Cook Time 20 minutes

Servings 2

Ingredients

- ½ tablespoon of extra virgin olive oil
- 1 avocado
- ¼ teaspoon of crushed red pepper chili flakes
- 1 large sweet potato
- 4 large eggs
- ¼ teaspoon of garlic salt

Directions:

1. First, you heat the oven to 375°F.
2. Then, while the oven is heating, cut sweet potato into four quarter-inch thick slices with a very sharp knife.
3. After which you line a baking sheet with parchment paper and place the four sweet potato slices on the paper.

4. After that, drizzle with olive oil over the sweet potatoes to evenly coat.
5. At this point, transfer to the oven and bake for 20 minutes, or until soft and slightly browned.
6. Furthermore, while the sweet potatoes are baking, bring 6 cups of water to a boil in a medium-sized pot.
7. Then, once the water is boiling, carefully place eggs into the pot and let boil for exactly 6 minutes.
8. This is when you slice the avocado in half and spoon into a small bowl, discarding the pit.
9. After that, add the garlic, sea salt and smash lightly with a fork.
10. In addition, once the eggs are done, carefully peel the shell under cold running water.
11. After which you assemble on a plate using the sweet potato as the toast.
12. Finally, spread avocado mash onto the toast, top with soft-boiled eggs, and garnish with crushed red pepper chili flakes.

Wholesome Cabbage Soup with Spicy Kimchi

Tips:

The mixture of fresh garlic, soy sauce, ginger, and sesame oil make this healthy cabbage soup like a stir-fry comfort food (only in hearty soup form).

Secondly, browning a little ground pork also makes it a filling main meal.

Course Main Course

Prep Time 10 minutes

Cook Time 25 minutes

Servings 4 people

Ingredients

- 1 medium yellow onion (chopped)
- 2 cloves garlic (minced)
- 4 cups of shredded cabbage (1 large head)
- 1 teaspoon of fish sauce
- 14 ounces' spicy kimchi (juice and all)
- 2 scallions (thinly sliced)
- 2 tablespoons of olive oil
- ½ pound ground pork
- 2 inches' ginger (minced)
- 2 tablespoons of soy sauce

1 teaspoon of toasted sesame oil

4 cups of Kettle and Fire Chicken Bone Broth

Directions

1. First, in a large pot over medium heat, warm the olive oil.
2. After which you add the onion and cook until translucent, 4 to 6 minutes.
3. After that, add the ground pork and cook, breaking it up with a spoon, until browned, 8 to 10 minutes.
4. Then, add the garlic and ginger and cook for another minute.
5. At this point, add the cabbage; then stir in the fish sauce, soy sauce, and sesame oil.
6. This is when you add the bone broth and bring to a boil.
7. Furthermore, reduce the heat to a simmer and cook, covered, until the cabbage is completely soft, 15 to 20 minutes.
8. After which you remove from the heat.
9. Finally, stir in the kimchi and kimchi juice.
10. You can serve and garnish with the scallions.

Recipe Notes

Remember to successfully preserve all the live active cultures in the kimchi, it's best to add it off heat, after the rest of soup has cooked.

COLLAGEN KETO RECIPES

Korean Keto Meatballs

Tips:

These recipe is keto-friendly taste like authentic Korean dumplings, without the added carbs.

Make sure you serve over sauteed cabbage and mushrooms for a complete, Asian-inspired dish.

Course Appetizer, Main Course

Prep Time 5 minutes

Cook Time 20 minutes

Servings 8

Ingredients

Ingredients for the meatballs:

- 1 white onion (finely chopped)
- 2 Tablespoons of toasted sesame oil
- Olive oil (for cooking)
- *2 lb. of ground pork*
- ¼ cup + 2 Tablespoons of coconut aminos
- 1 cup of green cabbage shredded
- ¼ teaspoon of black pepper

Ingredients for the sauce:

- 1 cup Kettle and Fire Chicken Bone Broth
- 2 Tablespoons of freshly grated ginger

1 can full-fat coconut milk

2 Tablespoons of coconut aminos

Directions:

1. Meanwhile, heat your oven to 400 degrees Fahrenheit.
2. After which in a large bowl, prepare your meatball mixture.
3. After that, combine onion, ground pork, coconut aminos, and sesame oil and mix; let sit for five minutes.
4. Furthermore, while your meatball mixture rests, prepare your sauce.
5. At this point, you whisk together chicken bone broth, coconut milk, coconut aminos, and fresh ginger in a pot over medium heat.
6. This is when you allow to cook for 5 minutes, then remove from heat.
7. In addition, return to your meatball mixture. Add the cabbage, and mix again.
8. After which you heat a cast iron skillet over medium-high heat; drizzle with olive oil.
9. After that, form your meatballs into small balls, roughly 1 to 1.5 inches in diameter.
10. Then, place into the cast skillet; sear for roughly 2 minutes, flip, then sear for another 2 minutes.
11. At this point, turn off the burner, and pour the sauce mixture directly into the cast iron pan with the meatballs.
12. Finally, transfer the entire pan to the oven; cook the meatballs for an additional 15 minutes, until cooked thoroughly.
13. Serve.

Loaded Cauliflower Keto Soup

Course Soup

Prep Time 5 minutes

Cook Time 20 minutes

Servings 8

Ingredients

- 1 Tablespoon of extra virgin olive oil
- 3 Tablespoons of minced garlic
- ½ teaspoon of red chili flakes
- 4 cups Kettle and Fire beef bone broth
- 2 cups of heavy cream
- Sour cream (for garnish)
- 8 strips of bacon
- 1 sweet onion (chopped)
- 1 Tablespoons of onion salt
- 3 Tablespoons of fresh chives
- 2 heads of cauliflower florets
- Green onions (for garnish)
- Shredded cheddar cheese (for garnish)

Directions:

1. First, heat a large cast iron pan or skillet over medium-high heat.
2. After which you place the bacon in the pan, cooking until crispy, or roughly two minutes per side; Set aside.
3. Then, while the bacon is cooking, heat a large soup pot or Dutch oven medium heat.
4. After that, drizzle olive oil in the pot, then add the chopped onion.
5. At this point, add the onion salt, garlic, red chili flakes, and chives to the large pot with the onion.
6. Furthermore, when the onion is translucent, but not caramelized, add the beef bone broth.
7. Add the cauliflower florets, and cover; cook for 15 minutes, or until fork-tender.
8. In addition, while the cauliflower is simmering, prepare your garnishes.
9. After which you chop the bacon and green onion.
10. After that, remove the cauliflower from heat, carefully pouring into a high-powered blender or food processor.
11. Then, blend in batches, as only half the mixture will fit into your food processor at one time.
12. At this point, hold tightly to the lid, as the heat will cause excessive pressure while blending; once fully blended, return the cauliflower mixture to the soup pot, turning the burner back to medium heat.
13. This is when, you stir in the heavy cream and bacon bits, reserving some bacon to be used as a garnish; continue to cook for 5 minutes.
14. Finally, pour soup into serving bowls and top with green onions, bacon, cheddar cheese, and sour cream.
15. Serve.

Creamy Keto Mushroom Soup

Tips:

1. This recipe will give you the same comfort food feeling that the old stuff did, but without all the carbs.
2. I bet after taking this recipe you will feel full from the heavy cream and mushroom fiber, and you'll get 10 grams of protein per serving from the bone broth as well — a balanced, low-carb soup that will satisfy the whole family.

Course Soup

Prep Time 5 minutes

Cook Time 15 minutes

Ingredients

1 leek (chopped and separated into green and white)

8 oz. mixed mushrooms diced (NOTE: we used a container that included: alba and brown clamshell, forest nameko, trumpet royale, velvet pioppini, and maitake frondosa)

1 ½ cups of Kettle and Fire Chicken Bone Broth

1 ½ cups of organic heavy cream (or better still full-fat coconut milk if going dairy-free)

2 Tablespoons of grass-fed butter + more for sautéing

2 cloves garlic (minced)

3 teaspoons of tamari

3 teaspoons of apple cider vinegar

Directions:

1. First, heat a large saucepan over medium heat until warm.

2. After which you melt 2 tablespoons butter and add the white part of the chopped leeks.
3. After that, sauté until translucent, then add garlic, stirring to make sure nothing burns.
4. Then, add mushrooms, stirring to coat everything with butter and allowing the aromas to release (about 3 minutes).
5. At this point, add tamari and chicken broth and continue stirring for another minute to marry all the flavors.
6. This is when you turn the heat down to low and scoop three fourths of the contents of the pot into a high-speed blender, leaving the other one fourth still in the saucepan.
7. Furthermore, blend until completely smooth and uniform.
8. Finally, return the blended soup to the pot and stir in the apple cider vinegar and heavy cream.

Optional: Add black pepper and additional tamari to taste.

Directions for the topping:

1. First, heat a separate large pot or skillet to medium heat.
2. After which you add a small pat of butter and the green portion of the chopped leeks.
3. After that, sauté until well-cooked and add a pinch of salt to taste.
4. Finally, top piping-hot soup with leek greens to your liking.

Instant Pot Spicy Creamy Keto Chicken Soup

Tip:

This recipe is made with nutrient-packed bone broth and tasty celery root, this keto chicken soup is comforting yet totally in line with keto requirements.

Course Soup

Prep Time 10 minutes

Cook Time 20 minutes

Ingredients

- 1 pound of chicken thigh or better still chicken breast
- 3 cloves garlic (peeled and pressed)
- 2 cups of Kettle and Fire Chicken Bone Broth
- 1 red bell pepper (chopped)
- 3 ribs celery (chopped)
- 1 jalapeno minced (NOTE: keep seeds for added spice or discard for mild)
- Salt and pepper (to taste)
- 1 Tablespoon of extra virgin olive oil
- ½ onion (chopped)
- 2 inches of ginger (peeled and minced)
- 1 celery root/celeriac cubed
- 2 large carrots (chopped)
- 3 oz. oyster mushrooms (chopped)

4 Tablespoons of cream cheese

1 cup of heavy cream

Optional Toppings:

3-5 scallions (finely chopped)

¼ avocado

Directions:

1. First, set the Instant Pot to high pressure at 10 minutes.
2. Then, when the pot is hot, add olive oil and chicken thighs.
3. After which you brown the chicken and add garlic, onion, and ginger, stirring until aromatic (about 2 minutes).
4. After that, add chicken broth and celery root and close lid.
5. Then, cook on high pressure for 10 minutes and allow steam to release naturally for another 10 minutes.
6. At this point, remove chicken, shred using a fork, and then place back into cooker.
7. This is when you add in remaining vegetables, except the optional scallions, and replace the Instant Pot lid.
8. Furthermore, set the timer to ZERO by pressing the "pressure cook" button and then pressing the "-" sign until it reaches "0." (This re-pressurizes the pot.)
9. After which you use the quick release valve to release the pressure.
10. In addition, remove lid and stir in heavy cream and cream cheese.
11. Finally, top with optional toppings and serve piping hot.

Homemade Keto Eggnog

Tip:

You can make a batch of this festive, holiday keto eggnog to enjoy with friends and family, no matter how you choose to celebrate. Cheers!

Course Drinks

Prep Time 20 minutes

Chill time 30 minutes

Servings 8 servings

Ingredients

- 2 cups of heavy cream (or better still full-fat coconut milk)
- 1/3 cup of Swerve
- 2 ounces' bourbon or to taste (it is optional)
- 4 eggs
- 1 cup of heavy whipping cream (or better still other non-dairy milk)
- 1 teaspoon of nutmeg

Directions:

1. First, using two large mixing bowls, separate the egg yolks from the egg whites; set the bowl with the egg whites aside.
2. Then, with a hand mixer, beat the egg yolks until they become a light, yellow color.
3. After which you gradually add in the Swerve until dissolved.
4. After that, add the heavy cream, heavy whipping cream, and nutmeg until well combined.

5. Furthermore, in a separate bowl, beat the egg whites until soft, white peaks form.
6. At this point, fold the egg whites into the egg yolk mixture; Chill.
7. Finally, right before serving, add the bourbon and lightly stir.
8. Make sure you serve with a sprinkle of nutmeg and cinnamon sticks.

Keto Fat Bombs with Cacao and Cashew

Tip:

1. This recipe in addition to being keto-friendly, they're also paleo, vegan, gluten-free, and dairy-free.
2. You can make this recipe your own by adding a dash of high quality, sugar-free vanilla extract, or a pinch of sea salt.

Course Snack

Prep Time 15 minutes

Cook Time 5 minutes

Servings 20 fat bombs

Ingredients

   1 cup of Almond Butter

   1 cup of Raw Cashews

   1 cup of Coconut Oil

   ¼ cup of Coconut Flour

   ½ cup of Cacao Powder

Directions:

1. First, in a non-stick medium saucepan over medium heat, heat coconut oil, and almond butter until mixed evenly, stirring often.
2. After which you pour the oil mixture from the pan into a bowl and mix in coconut flour and cacao powder.
3. After that, place bowl in the freezer for about 15 minutes until mixture cools and is solid.
4. Then, while the mixture is cooling, place the cashews in a food processor and pulse lightly for a chopped texture.

5. At this point, when the coconut mixture is solidified, take ½ tablespoon of the mixture from the bowl, roll into a ball, and dip in the blended cashews.
6. This is when you place fat bombs on a plate.
7. Furthermore, repeat until you have used all of the mixture.
8. Finally, refrigerate the fat bombs for 5 minutes.

NOTE: Enjoy and make sure to store your leftover fat bombs in the refrigerator, otherwise they will melt quickly.

Keto Broccoli Cheese Soup

Tips:

This recipe is a keto-approved comfort food that's sure to satisfy your taste buds—and your macros.

Course Soup

Prep Time 5 minutes

Cook Time 32 minutes

Servings 4 people

Ingredients

- ½ onion (diced)
- 3 celery stalks (chopped)
- 4 cups broccoli florets (chopped)
- 2 cups of heavy whipping cream organic
- 3 cups of sharp cheddar cheese shredded
- 2 strips of uncured bacon
- 3 carrot sticks (chopped)
- 5 cloves garlic (minced)
- 2 cups of Kettle and Fire Chicken Bone Broth
- ¼ teaspoon of Himalayan pink salt
- ¼ teaspoon of black pepper ground

Directions:

1. First, in a large pot over medium heat, cook the bacon until brown and crispy, about 2 minutes each side.

2. After which you remove the bacon from the pot and set aside.
3. After that, keep the bacon grease in the pot and add the carrots, onions, celery, and garlic.
4. Then, let cook for 10 minutes, stirring occasionally.
5. Furthermore, once the vegetables are tender, add the broccoli, chicken bone broth, heavy whipping cream, salt and pepper to the pot.
6. This is when you bring to a simmer and cook for 10 minutes.
7. In addition, slowly stir in the cheddar cheese, allowing it to melt into the soup.
8. At this point, once all the cheese has been incorporated, cook for 10 minutes.
9. Finally, while the soup simmers, roughly chop the bacon strips.
10. You can divide soup into 4 servings and garnish with bacon bits and any remaining cheese.

Keto Brussels Sprouts Gratin

Tip:

This recipe is full of keto-friendly fats to help you meet your macros, satisfy your appetite, and stay in ketosis over the holidays.

Course Side Dish

Prep Time 10 minutes

Cook Time 25 minutes

Servings 4

Ingredients

- 1 large shallot (minced)
- ½ pound Brussels sprouts finely shredded or better still quartered
- 1 cup of organic heavy cream
- Kosher salt
- ¼ cup of pine nuts (finely chopped)
- 2 tablespoons of grated parmesan cheese
- 2 tablespoons of olive oil
- 2 cloves garlic (minced)
- 1 cup Kettle and Fire Mushroom Chicken Bone Broth
- 1 cup of organic mozzarella cheese shredded
- 1 pinch nutmeg
- 4 sprigs thyme leaves (finely chopped)

Directions:

1. First, in a large sauce pot over medium heat, warm the olive oil.
2. After which you add the shallots and garlic and cook, stirring, until just soft, 2 to 3 minutes.
3. After that, add the Brussels sprouts and stir to combine.
4. At this point, add the bone broth to the pot and stir to combine.
5. Then, cook until the Brussels sprouts are just soft, 3 to 5 minutes; stir in the heavy cream and cheese.
6. This is when you add the nutmeg and a couple generous pinches of salt.
7. Furthermore, cook until cheese it completely melted, 1 to 2 minutes.
8. In the meantime, in a small bowl, combine the pine nuts, thyme and parmesan cheese.
9. Add a pinch of salt and toss gently to combine; carefully divide the Brussels sprouts and cream mixture evenly between the four ramekins and top with the pine nut mixture.
10. After that, place ramekins on a sheet pan and transfer to the oven.
11. Then, cook until the gratin is bubbly and the pine nut crust is golden brown, 10 to 12 minutes.
12. Finally, remove from the oven, let cool slightly and serve.

Keto Pizza with Pepperoni

Tips:

Sometimes we can't believe the keto diet is called a diet, especially when you get your hands on recipes like this Keto Pizza with Pepperoni.

Course Main Course

Prep Time 10 minutes

Cook Time 20 minutes

Servings 2

Ingredients

For the pizza crust:

- 1 ½ cups of organic mozzarella cheese whole milk
- 2 large eggs
- 2 tablespoons of organic cream cheese full-fat
- ⅓ cup of coconut flour

Ingredients for the toppings:

- ½ cup of organic mozzarella cheese whole milk
- 8 slices of pepperoni uncured
- ¼ cup of sugar-free marinara sauce

Directions:

To make the pizza crust:

1. Meanwhile, heat oven to 425°F.

2. After which you line a baking sheet with parchment paper. (NOTE: Do not substitute for tin foil as dough will stick.)
3. After that, add 1 ½ cups of mozzarella cheese and 2 tablespoons cream cheese to a microwave safe, medium size bowl.
4. Then, microwave on medium heat for 90 seconds, stirring the ingredients in the bowl halfway through to properly melt all ingredients.
5. Furthermore, stir in coconut flour and 2 large eggs into the bowl and mix thoroughly with a fork.
6. At this point, you knead with your hands until mixture becomes dough, about 2 minutes.
7. In addition, with your hands spread the dough on the baking sheet, creating a round shape giving the crust about ¼-inch thickness.
8. Finally, using a fork, poke holes into crust all over multiple times to avoid bubbles; bake for 10 minutes.

Directions to assemble the pizza:

1. First, you spread ¼ cup sugar-free marinara sauce onto the crust creating an even layer.
2. After which you sprinkle the remaining ½ cup of mozzarella cheese onto the pizza.
3. After that, place 8 slices of pepperoni evenly.
4. Then, return the pizza back to the oven for 10 more minutes or until the crust edges and cheese toppings are golden brown.

Baked Almond-Crusted Cod with Sautéed Bok Choy and Bell Peppers

Tip:

1. This recipe is SIBO-friendly, it simple a collection of flavors combined to create something greater than the sum of its parts.
2. A white fish (we prefer Rock Cod, but any white fish will do), stone ground mustard, fresh garden herbs, and a bed of SIBO-friendly vegetables are all plated beautifully and packed with flavor.

Course Main Course

Prep Time 10 minutes

Cook Time 10 minutes

Servings 4 people

Ingredients

- 2 sprigs parsley leaves (minced)
- ¼ cup stone ground (mustard)
- sea salt
- 4 tablespoons of avocado oil
- 2 red bell peppers (thinly sliced)
- ½ cup of slivered almonds (roughly chopped)
- 2 sprigs rosemary leaves (minced)
- 2 sprigs oregano leaves (minced)
- 2 tablespoons of apple cider vinegar

Freshly ground black pepper

1 ¼ pounds fresh Rock Cod filets (or better still your favorite white fish)

6 baby bok choy stems and leaves separated and coarsely chopped

1 lemon (sliced into wedges)

Directions:

1. First, heat oven to 350°F.
2. After which in a small bowl, mix half the mustard, herbs, apple cider vinegar, and a pinch of salt and pepper until all ingredients are fully incorporated.
3. After that, grease a 9 x 13-inch baking dish or pan with 1 tablespoon of avocado oil and place the fish on top.
4. Then, spread an even layer of the mustard mixture over the top of each fillet.
5. At this point, evenly distribute slivered almonds on top of each fillet.
6. This is when you drizzle a thin layer of avocado oil and another pinch of salt over the almonds.
7. Furthermore, transfer to the oven and bake until the fish is flakey and opaque, about 10 minutes.
8. Then broil for about 2 minutes to brown slightly; quickly remove from the oven.
9. After that, in a large frying pan over medium-high heat, warm 2 tablespoons of avocado oil.
10. In addition, add pepper and bok choy stems and cook, stirring, until softened, about 2 minutes.
11. After which you add the bok choy leaves and cook until wilted, about 1 minute.

12. At this point, remove from the heat and stir in a few generous pinches of salt and pepper.
13. Finally, plate in large bowls with the veggies on the bottom with the fish on top.
14. Spoon the juices from the baking dish over the fish and garnish with a slice of lemon and remaining fresh chopped herbs.

Keto Overnight Oats with Coconut and Blueberries

Tip:

This recipe contains healthy fats, fiber, and flavor; you won't even notice the oats are missing!

Course Breakfast

Prep Time 5 minutes

Cook Time 4 hours

Servings 1

Ingredients

- 2 tablespoons of pecans (roughly chopped)
- 1 teaspoon of cinnamon ground
- 2 tablespoons of water
- 10 blueberries for garnish
- 6 tablespoons of hemp hearts
- 2 teaspoons of chia seeds
- 5 tablespoons of full-fat coconut milk
- ½ teaspoon of erythritol or better still 3 drops liquid stevia, optional for sweetness

Directions:

1. First, in an 8-ounce mason jar, mix in all the ingredients (minus the blueberries) with a spoon until thoroughly combined.
2. After which you place in the refrigerator overnight, or for a minimum of 4 hours.
3. Finally, garnish with blueberries and enjoy.

The Best Keto Meatloaf

Tip:

This recipe is juicy, flavor-packed; topped with a tangy and sweet tomato sauce that is gluten-free and low carb to meet your keto diet needs.

Course Main Course

Prep Time 15 minutes

Cook Time 55 minutes

Servings 6 slices

Ingredients

Ingredients for the meatloaf:

- 2 large cage-free eggs
- 2 cloves garlic (minced)
- 1 teaspoon of coconut aminos
- ¼ cup of unsweetened almond milk
- 1 tablespoon of dried oregano
- 1 teaspoon of ground black pepper
- 1 ½ pounds of ground beef
- 1 small onion (diced)
- 2 cups mushrooms (finely chopped)
- 1 tablespoon of tomato paste
- ¼ cup of almond flour
- 1 teaspoon of Himalayan pink salt

Ingredients for the tomato sauce:

½ teaspoon of Himalayan pink salt

½ teaspoon of dried oregano

1 heirloom tomato sliced, (it is optional)

1 cup of tomatoes (diced)

½ teaspoon of ground black pepper

½ teaspoon of dried parsley

Directions:

1. First, heat oven to 350°F.
2. After which in a large bowl, combine all the meatloaf ingredients and knead the mixture with your hands until fully combined.
3. After that, in a non-stick, 9x5-inch loaf pan, add the meatloaf mixture and press down to fill all the edges of the pan; set aside.
4. Then, in a small pot over low heat, add the tomato sauce ingredients and bring to a simmer.
5. At this point, cook for 2 minutes, stirring occasionally.
6. This is when you remove from the heat and pour the tomato sauce over the meatloaf. (you can add slices of heirloom tomato to garnish).
7. Furthermore, place in the oven and cook until the meatloaf is cooked through and no longer pink in the middle, about 50 minutes.
8. Finally, remove from the oven and let rest until warm, about 10 minutes. Serve.

Keto Fried Chicken

This recipe is fried in tallow and coated with a gluten-free, Southern-spiced batter, this keto fried chicken has the crunch you've been craving.

Course Main Course

Prep Time 5 minutes

Cook Time 40 minutes

Servings 2 people

Ingredients

- ½ tablespoon of cayenne pepper
- ½ tablespoon of dried oregano
- 1 teaspoon of black pepper
- 2 chicken thighs skin on
- ¼ cup of tallow (rendered suet)
- 1 cup of almond flour
  - ½ tablespoon of garlic powder
- 1 teaspoon of salt
- 1 egg
- 2 chicken drumsticks skin on

Directions:

1. First, in a medium bowl, add the cayenne pepper, dried oregano, flour, garlic powder, salt and pepper. Mix with a fork until fully blended.
2. After which you spread the mixture on a large flat plate.

3. Then, in another small bowl, crack the egg and beat with a fork.
4. Furthermore, one by one, dip the chicken in the bowl with the egg until fully coated.
5. After which you dredge each chicken piece in the flour and spice mixture on the plate until all sides are fully coated; repeat with all the chicken.
6. After that, in a large saucepan over medium heat, warm the tallow until melted.
7. Then, once the tallow is melted and bubbling, add the chicken. (You should hear a sizzle as soon as it hits the pan.)
8. At this point, fry the chicken, flipping once, until golden brown, about 10 minutes on either side.
9. This is when you cover the pan with a lid, lower the heat, and cook until the chicken is no longer pink in the middle, about 20 minutes. (NOTE: Fully cooked chicken should be 165°F in the thickest part.)
10. Finally, transfer the chicken to a paper towel-lined plate to let the grease drip off.
11. Make sure you enjoy with a side salad or sautéed vegetables.

COLLAGEN SMOOTHIE AND SHAKES

Creamy Chocolate Collagen Smoothie

Prep time: 10 minutes

Yield: 2 servings

Ingredients:

- 2 frozen bananas
- 2 cups OF unsweetened almond milk (or preferably coconut milk)
- 1 avocado
- ½ cup of frozen raspberries (or better still fresh raspberries or other berries)
- 2 scoops of Cob Ionic Indulgence (Chocolate Collagen)

Direction:

1. First, add all ingredients to your blender and blend until smooth.
2. Then, pour into glasses, decorate with raspberries and coconut flakes.

Blueberry Explosion Collagen Smoothie

Prep time: 10 minutes

Yield: 2 servings

Ingredients:

- ½ cup of blueberries
- 2 scoops of Cob Ionic Indulgence (Chocolate Collagen)
- 1 cup of unsweetened almond milk (or better still coconut milk)
- ½ cup ice

Directions:

1. First, add all ingredients to your blender and blend until smooth.
2. Then, pour into a mason jar and decorate with colorful paper straws.

Chocolate Almond Butter Collagen Shake

Prep time: 10 minutes

Yield: 2 servings

Ingredients:

- 1 scoop of Cob Ionic Indulgence (Chocolate Collagen)
- ¼ cup ice
- 1 cup of unsweetened almond milk (or better still coconut milk)
- 1 Tablespoon of almond butter
- 1 teaspoon of vanilla extract

Directions:

1. First, add all ingredients to your blender and blend until smooth.
2. Then, pour into glasses and enjoy!

Chocolate Peppermint Collagen Smoothie

Prep time: 10 minutes

Yield: 2 servings

Ingredients:

- 1 small avocado
- 2 scoops of Cob Ionic Indulgence (Chocolate Collagen)
- ½ teaspoon of peppermint extract
- 2 cups of unsweetened almond milk (or better still coconut milk)
- 1 cup ice

Directions:

1. First, add all ingredients to your blender and blend until completely smooth.
2. Then, pour into glasses and garnish with fresh peppermint leaves.

Chocolate Peppermint Collagen Smoothie

Prep time: 10 minutes

Yield: 2 servings

Ingredients:

- 1 small avocado
- ½ teaspoon of peppermint extract
- 2 cups of unsweetened almond milk (or better still coconut milk)
- 1 cup ice
- 2 scoops of Cob Ionic Indulgence (Chocolate Collagen)

Directions:

1. First, add all ingredients to your blender and blend until completely smooth.
2. Then, pour into glasses and garnish with fresh peppermint leaves.

Acai Superfood Collagen Smoothie

Prep time: 5 minutes

Yield: 2 servings

Ingredients:

- 1 cup (about 80g) frozen raspberries
- ½ scoop of Cob Ionic Indulgence (Chocolate Collagen)
- 1 packet (about 100g) frozen, unsweetened acai puree
- 1 small frozen banana
- 1 cup of unsweetened almond milk (or better still coconut milk)
- **Optional:** Handful of berries, 1 teaspoon of poppy seeds, 1 teaspoon of shredded coconut for topping

Directions:

1. First, add all ingredients to your blender and blend until completely smooth.
2. Then, pour into glasses and garnish with toppings (optional).

German Chocolate Cake Collagen Smoothie

Prep time: 10 minutes

Yield: 2 servings

Ingredients:

- 2 scoops of Cob Ionic Indulgence (Chocolate Collagen)
- 1 cup of crushed ice
- 1 teaspoon of chopped pecans
- 2 cups of dairy-free milk
- 1 small avocado
- 1 teaspoon of unsweetened shredded coconut

It is Optional: Chopped pecans, 100% dark chocolate, grated and unsweetened shredded coconut for topping

Directions:

1. First, add all the smoothie ingredients to your blender and blend until completely smooth.
2. Then, pour into glasses and garnish with chopped pecans, grated 100% dark chocolate and unsweetened shredded coconut.

Chocolate Mint Shake

Course Breakfast, Dessert

Ingredients

- ¼ cup of avocado
- 1 to 2 tablespoons of raw honey (to taste)
- 6 to 8 dried peppermint fresh
- ½ cup ice cubes made from pure water
- 8 ounces' full fat coconut milk or any other raw or non-dairy milk
- 1 to 2 tablespoons of cacao powder
- 1 tablespoon of sustainably sourced collagen
- 1 to 2 tablespoons of allergy-friendly chocolate chips optional, but yummy!

Directions:

1. First, combine ingredients in the order listed in a blender.
2. Then, blend until smooth and enjoy!

Best Keto Collagen Peptide Smoothie Ever (Easy Recipe)

Prep Time: 5 minutes

Total Time: 5 minutes

Ingredients

1 ½ teaspoon of chia seeds

1 scoop (1/3 oz.) collagen peptides

½ cup of unsweetened almond milk

¼ – ½ cup ice

¼ large avocado

1 tablespoon of cocoa powder

1 tablespoon of almond butter

½ cup of water

liquid stevia to taste (it is optional)

Directions:

1. First, place all the ingredients in a blender and blend until smooth.
2. Serve immediately.

Strawberry Moringa Mint Smoothie

Prep Time: 10 minutes

Serves: 2

Ingredients:

- 1.5 cup of full fat unsweetened coconut
- ¼ cup of fresh mint (feel free to substitute ¼ teaspoon organic peppermint oil)
- 1 cup of frozen cauliflower rice
- 1 tablespoon of Brain Octane oil (15% off now)
- 1.5 cup of frozen strawberries
- 1 tablespoon of chia seeds (soaked in blender with milk for 10 min)
- ½ stevia powder (or better still 15-20 drops liquid stevia)
- 1 tablespoon of moringa powder (I use Kuli Kuli)
- optional: 1 scoop vanilla protein powder, 1-2 tablespoons collagen, vanilla extract, turmeric, cinnamon, and/or coconut butter

Directions for smoothie:

1. First, add coconut milk and chia seeds to the blender and let soak for 10 minutes.
2. After which you put the rest of the ingredients in blender and blend.
3. Then, top with mint and moringa to make it extra pretty.

Note: Do not blend collagen in, all you do is just pulse to mix.

Blueberry Muffin Smoothie Bowl Healthy Recipe

INGREDIENTS:

1 scoop vanilla protein powder

1 cup of plain, nonfat Greek yogurt

1 tablespoon of honey

1 cup ice

2 cups of unsweetened almond milk

1 ½ cups of fresh blueberries

¾ cup of old-fashioned oats

½ teaspoon of vanilla extract

½ teaspoons of sea salt

Directions:

1. First, place all of the ingredients in a blender and process until smooth.
2. Then, pour into 2 bowls and sprinkle with a few oats and blueberries.
3. Enjoy with a spoon.

Blueberry Muffin Smoothie Bowl

Course   Breakfast

Servings

Ingredients

- 1 scoop vanilla protein powder
- 1 cup plain, nonfat Greek yogurt
- 1 tablespoon of honey
- 1 cup ice
- 2 cups of unsweetened almond milk
- 1 ½ cups of fresh blueberries
- ¾ cup of old-fashioned oats
- ½ teaspoon of vanilla extract

Directions:

1. First, place all of the ingredients in a blender and process until smooth.
2. Then, pour into 2 bowls and sprinkle with a few oats and blueberries.
3. Enjoy with a spoon.

Apple Banana Smoothie

Course: Drinks

Prep Time: 5 minutes

Cook Time: 2 minutes

Servings: 2 servings

A simply delicious apple banana smoothie filled with nutrients.

Ingredients

- 5.3 ounces Plain Greek yogurt (whole milk)
- 1 banana
- ¼ teaspoon of vanilla
- 2 Tablespoons of protein powder optional
- 6 oz. black brewed tea (I prefer English Breakfast Tea)
- 1 apple
- 2 Tablespoons of peanut butter
- ⅛ teaspoon of cinnamon (for topping)

Directions:

1. First, brew 6 ounces of black tea (NOTE: I prefer English Breakfast Tea). Chill tea.
2. After which you peel, core and slice apple into pieces.
3. After that, peel and cut a banana into pieces.
4. Then, place all the ingredients in a blender and puree until smooth.
5. At this point, pour into two 8-ounce glasses.
6. This is when, you sprinkle with cinnamon.

7. Then, add a straw and serve.

Yields 16 ounces.

Raw Superfood Smoothie

Prep Time: 5 minutes

Cook Time: 0 minutes

Servings: 4

Ingredients

1 ripe banana

1 teaspoon of mesquite powder (or better still maca)

A splash of water

1 teaspoon of blackstrap molasses

5 soft pitted dates

4 – 5 frozen bananas

1 teaspoon of vanilla extract

1 tablespoon of cacao nibs

Directions:

1. First, put the water, dates, vanilla, mesquite powder and 1 ripe banana in a blender and process until smooth.
2. After which you add chunks of frozen bananas slowly until you have smooth ice-cream.
3. After that, transfer into a large glass jar or bowl and sprinkle with nibs and drizzle on the molasses.

NOTE: it may get a bit messy but just roll with it.

4. Then, blackstrap molasses is an acquired taste but super healthy.

Steamed Spinach Smoothie "Pucks"

Ingredients

½ cup of pure water

1/3 cup of measuring cup

36 ounces washed fresh baby spinach

1 cookie sheet

unbleached parchment paper

Directions:

1. First, line cookie sheet with unbleached parchment paper.
2. After which you prepare to steam the spinach. (**NOTE:** I do not have a special steamer or steaming basket. I simply place a stainless steel colander inside of a larger pot with a bit of boiling water in the bottom)
3. After that, place as much spinach as will fit into your steamer (or better still pot + colander over boiling water).
4. Then, cover the spinach and steam for 1 minute.
5. At this point, remove from the heat; pack the steamed spinach into the measuring cup.
6. This is when you flip it over and give it a tap onto the parchment-lined cookie sheet. (NOTE: It should come out the same size and shape as the measuring cup).
7. Furthermore, continue to do this until all the spinach has been used.
8. After which you place the cookie sheet into the freezer.
9. In addition, freeze 4 to 6 hours, or until the spinach is in solid "pucks".
10. After that, store in a zip-top bag in the freezer.
11. Finally, add 1 smoothie puck to any smoothie for a boost of good-for-you greens with lots of absorbable calcium!

Roasted Strawberry Protein Smoothie

Prep Time: 3 mins

Cook Time: 12 mins

Course: Breakfast, Brunch, Snack

Tip:

This recipe is made with creamy cottage cheese and added chia seeds – what a great way to start the day!

Ingredients

- ½ tablespoon of raw sugar
- ½ cup of fat free milk
- 6 to 8 drops liquid stevia (it is optional)
- 1-1/2 cups of fresh strawberries (quartered)
- 1/3 cup of reduced fat cottage cheese
- 1 cup of crushed ice
- 1 teaspoon of chia seeds

Directions:

1. Meanwhile, heat oven to 425°F.
2. After which, in a medium bowl, combine strawberries and sugar.
3. After that, pour the strawberries on a parchment paper lined baking sheet.
4. Then, place in the oven and roast for 12 to 15 minutes until the strawberries start to release their juices but are still firm.

5. Finally, carefully pour the roasted strawberries and their juice into a blender along with milk, cottage cheese, ice and chia and blend until smooth.
6. Enjoy!

Keto Smoothie - Blueberry

Tips:

This recipe is perfect for a quick breakfast or a post-workout refuel option.

It's packed with vitamin c for a healthy immune system, antioxidants for better detoxification, and folate for proper cholesterol function.

Course Breakfast, Snack

Prep Time 5 minutes

Servings 1 Serving

Ingredients

- ¼ cup of Blueberries
- 30 g Protein Powder (it is optional)
- 1 cup of Coconut Milk (or better still almond milk)
- 1 teaspoon of Vanilla Extract
- 1 teaspoon of MCT Oil (or better still coconut oil)

Directions:

First, put all the ingredients into a blender, and blend until smooth.

Happy Digestion Smoothie

Tips:

1. This recipe is packed with digestion-enhancing and immune-boosting foods like parsley, pineapple, ginger, and avocado.
2. You can add a handful of baby spinach to boost the nutrient power even more.
3. In addition, fresh mint also gives this smoothie a nice digestion boost (not to mention a delicious minty flavor).
4. Remember, if you are averse to the spiciness of ginger, I suggest starting with half the amount and adding to taste from there and it also keeps well overnight.

Yield 2 1/4 cups (560 mL)

Prep time 10 Minutes

Cook time 0 Minutes

Ingredients:

½ large frozen banana

½ cup (about 125 mL) coconut water

2 tablespoons of avocado

lemon or lime slice (for garnish)

1 heaping cup frozen pineapple chunks

½ cup (about 125 mL) water

¼ cup of packed fresh parsley leaves

1 teaspoon of packed fresh grated ginger

¼ teaspoon of probiotic powder (optional)

Directions:

1. First, add all ingredients into a blender.
2. Blend on the highest speed until super smooth.

Kale Blueberry Smoothie

Ingredients:

3 frozen bananas

2 scoops of Sun warrior Classic + raw vegan protein in chocolate or better still vanilla

3-4 cups of water (or as needed)

10 large curly kale leaves (stems removed)

2 cups of frozen blueberries

2 Tablespoons of raw cacao nibs

Directions:

1. First, place greens and water at the bottom of your blender container.
2. After which you add protein powder, then remaining ingredients.
3. After that, blend until desired consistency is achieved, adding more water if needed.
4. Then, store in glass jars with plastic lids for best freshness. (**NOTE:** I prefer drinking this smoothie within 24 hours of making it).

Better Than Botox Green Smoothie

Serves: 1

Ingredients

- 1 large handful spinach
- 2 tablespoons of almond butter
- 2 dates
- 1 teaspoon of flaxseeds
- 4 frozen strawberries
- 1 cup of organic almond milk (NOTE: look for a carrageenan free brand like this)
- 2 leaves of kale (stems removed)
- 2 tablespoons of pumpkin seeds
- 1 teaspoon of cinnamon
- 1 frozen banana

Directions:

1. First, toss all ingredients into a blender and blend baby, blend.
2. Then, prepare yourself for endless compliments on your radiant, glowing skin.

Blueberry Granola Power Smoothie

Prep Time 5 mins

Course: Breakfast

Servings: 1 adult smoothie

Ingredients

- ¾ cup of Real California milk preferably whole
- ½ whole banana
- 1-2 tablespoons of raw honey
- ice
- ½ cup of Real California yogurt preferably whole fat
- 1 cup of frozen or fresh blueberries
- 2 tablespoons of granola
- 1 scoop collagen protein powder (optional)
- 1 tablespoon of chia seeds (optional)

Directions:

1. First, place all ingredients in the blender and process until very smooth.
2. Enjoy immediately.

Keto Chocolate Smoothie

Prep Time 5 mins

Course: Breakfast

Servings: 4

Ingredients

- 1 cup of canned coconut milk
- 3 tablespoons of unsweetened cocoa powder
- 3 tablespoons of Swerve Confectioners or better still sweetener of choice
- Ice (optional)
- 2 cups of plain almond milk
- ½ avocado (optional)
- 2 tablespoons of collagen protein
- 1 tablespoon of MCT oil
- 1 teaspoon of vanilla extract

Directions:

1. First, place almond milk, avocado, Swerve, coconut milk, collagen protein, cocoa powder, MCT oil, and vanilla in a high speed blender.
2. After which you process until smooth.
3. Then, if desired add ice and process until crushed.

Banana Chocolate Collagen Shake

Course   Appetizer / Snack, Breakfast

Prep Time   5 minutes

Ingredients

- ½ cup of vanilla coconut yogurt (optional)
- 2 tablespoons of almond butter
- 2 scoops collagen peptides (I recommend Vital Proteins brand)
- 1 cup ice
- 1 cup of vanilla almond milk
- 1 medium ripe banana
- 1 tablespoon of organic cocoa powder
- ½ teaspoon of stevia

Directions:

1. First, place all ingredients into blender and process on high for 1 minute.
2. Then, pour into your favorite glass and enjoy!

Blueberry Collagen Smoothie

Prep Time: 5 minutes
Cook Time: 0 minutes
Yield: 1-2 servings 1x

Ingredients

½ frozen banana

1 tablespoon of almond butter

2 scoops of collagen powder (about 20 grams of collagen)

1 cup ice (optional)

1 cup of blueberries

½ ripe avocado

1 tablespoon of chia seeds

1 and ½ cups of milk of any kind or water (I use THIS)

Directions:

1. First, combine all ingredients in a blender and process until creamy smooth.
2. Enjoy!

Blueberry Collagen Smoothie (Glowing Skin!)

Prep Time: 5 mins

Total Time: 5 mins

Yield: 1 1x

Ingredients

1 scoop Vital Proteins Collagen Peptides Powder

1 Tablespoon of Cashew Butter

1 cup of Coconut Water

1 handful Blueberries

1 frozen Banana

Directions:

1. First, add all ingredients to a high speed blender and blend for 30 seconds until smooth and creamy.
2. Enjoy!

COOL AS A CUCUMBER SMOOTHIE

MAKES 1 SERVING

Ingredients:

1 cup of coconut water

½ cup of chopped papaya

Several ice cubes

1 medium cucumber (peeled, seeded, and chopped)

½ cup of chopped cantaloupe

1 small lemon (peeled, quartered, and seeded)

Directions:

1. First, in a blender, combine the coconut water, papaya, cucumber, cantaloupe, lemon, and ice cubes.
2. Then, blend until the desired consistency is reached. Serve ice cold.

NOTE: for best results, I recommend you chill all ingredients before preparing.

THE BRAZILIAN FACE-LIFT

MAKES 1 SERVING

Ingredients:

1 cup of chopped kale

2 Brazil nuts

1 cup of coconut water

1 cup of fresh (or better still frozen blueberries)

1 orange (peeled)

Directions:

1. First, in a blender, combine the kale, orange, coconut water, blueberries, and Brazil nuts.
2. Then, blend until the desired consistency is reached. Drink up!

ISLAND TIME SHIFTER

MAKES 1 SERVING

Ingredients:

1 cup of fresh or frozen chopped mango

½ cup of unsweetened coconut milk

10 almonds

1 cup of fresh or frozen strawberries

1 avocado

2 tablespoons of shredded unsweetened coconut, divided

Directions:

1. First, in a blender, combine the mango, coconut milk, avocado, strawberries, 1 tablespoon of the coconut, and the almonds.
2. Then, blend until the desired consistency is reached.
3. Finally, sprinkle the remaining 1 tablespoon shredded coconut on top of the smoothie and enjoy!

www.ingramcontent.com/pod-product-compliance
Lightning Source LLC
Chambersburg PA
CBHW081724100526
44591CB00016B/2490